How To Fix Of Your Thyroid Problems

"Discover Hidden Ideas That Fix Your Thyroid"

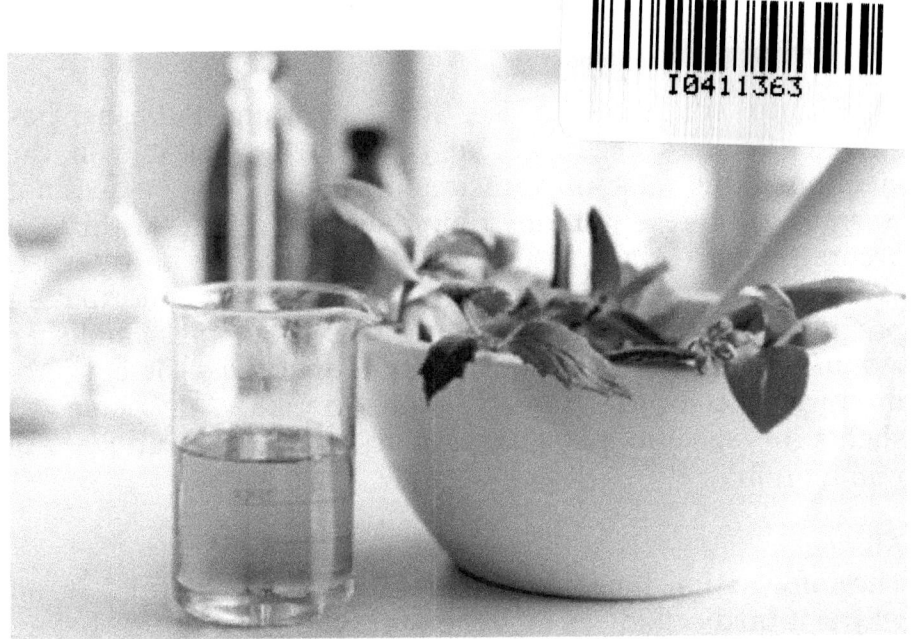

By Rudy S Silva, Natural Nutritionist

Table Of Contents

1: What to Expect From This Thyroid Book

Many people have thyroid problems or diseases and they don't know it. Many times you may go to a doctor not knowing what is wrong with you. The doctor, also, may have a hard time trying to figure out why you don't feel good.

If you have a thyroid issue, the doctor may not determine this right away, because many thyroid symptoms are also symptoms of other diseases.

Thyroid symptoms can be subtle and related to other diseases. These symptoms can take months or even years to develop and show up. When this is the case, it is difficult to attribute these symptoms to a thyroid condition.

This book is mostly concerned with hypothyroidism and hyperthyroidism. Other types of thyroid diseases are mention on occasion. The function of the thyroid is also covered and should be of benefit to all. By knowing how something works, you have a better chance of fixing it.

There are many thyroid diseases that occur such as an overactive or underactive thyroid, lump in the thyroid, or pregnancy thyroid. In this book, we detail what you need to do to overcome an unhealthy thyroid by outlining natural ways that you can improve the health of your thyroid.

If you have a cyst in your thyroid, the information here will help you to decrease its size by detoxifying your body. Other thyroid diseases that are more serious can also be helped with this information. But in cases where there has be irreparable tissue damage, surgery or other medical attention may be needed.

Thyroid Problem Symptoms

If you have an underactive thyroid, the symptoms associated with this condition are weight gain, fatigue, lack of energy, lack of patience, trouble concentrating, constipation, dry skin, thinning hair, feeling cold, high cholesterol, or restlessness, . These symptoms can lead to depression, over sensitive, argumentative, or loss of sex drive. Other symptoms may include,

Memory loss
Cold hands or feet
Inability to lose weight
Menstrual problems
Thinning hair
Migraines
Hypertension
Infertility

If you have an overactive thyroid, the some symptoms are nervousness, anxiety, insomnia, racing heartbeat, excess perspiration or weight loss. These symptoms can lead to other psychological issue.

A poor functioning thyroid can also create Alzheimer's like symptoms.

Thyroid Location

Your thyroid is right under your jaw and in front of your throat on top of your wind pipe. This position makes it easy to see lumps or cysts that develop in the thyroid. When you have a lump, you may have a hard time breathing or swallowing, if the lump gets too large.

When your thyroid enlarges, it's called goiter. This is a disease that is typically occurs from a lack of iodine and is found in many third world countries.

Thyroid Surgery

Doctors are quick to remove the thyroid, when there are signs of disease or certain conditions. The removal of the thyroid is life changing, since you will need to take medication for the rest of your life, to compensate for the lack of the thyroid hormone, thyroxine.

Your thyroid plays a major role your body's normal growth and function. It is critical for your mental and physical growth and health. It controls your body's metabolism, and, as such, provides all of your organs and cells with the energy they need to give your life.

2: Why Your Thyroid Gives You Problems

Thyrotropin

Your brain controls the secretions or release of the thyroid hormone. First, a thyrotropin releasing hormone, **TRH**, is released by your hypothalamus located in your brain. This hormone, **TRH,** acts as a messenger and tells your pituitary gland to release the thyroid-stimulating hormone, **TSH**.

The Thyroid-stimulating hormone, **TSH**, reaches the thyroid and stimulates it to release the thyroid hormone.

Thyroglobulin

Thyroglobulin is a protein that is created in your thyroid. When thyroglobulin and iodine combine, the thyroid hormone is created. Two forms of the thyroid hormone exist – Thyroxine, **T4**, and triiodothyronine, **T3** and when created in the thyroid, they are released into your blood stream. When the **T4** travels into certain organs and tissue, it is converted to **T3**. It is **T3** that does the final work in your cells and tissues to give you energy and life.

The secretions of your thyroid gland are controlled within your blood stream. When too much **T3 or T4** exist in your blood, a message is sent to your brain to reduce the amount of **TRH** and **TSH** being released. This helps to prevent an over active thyroid condition or hyperthyroidism.

When there is not enough **T3 or T4** in your blood, a message is sent to your brain to release more **TRH** and **TSH**. This helps to prevent an under active thyroid or hypothyroidism.

The thyroid gland can malfunction when the hypothalamus or pituitary gland are injured by disease or by trauma. An upset in the balance between the **TRH** and **TSH** causes an upset in the proper production of the thyroid hormone.

What Is Thyroxine And Tyrosine

Thyroxine, the hormone released by your thyroid, is composed of two molecules of tyrosine, where each molecule has attached to it two other molecules of an iodine compound. Tyrosine is called a nonessential amino acid that comes from protein. When you eat meat, you are getting tyrosine. However, since your body can make tyrosine from the amino acid phenylalanine, your body does not need you to provide it. You can still be short on tyrosine, if your body is not functioning properly.

One of the tyrosine functions is to help make and regulate hormones in the thyroid, adrenal, pituitary glands. It is also involved in being part of almost every protein in your body. So, you can see how important tyrosine is, since it is working with the pituitary and thyroid gland, which provides you with the right amount of Thyroxine.

The thyroxine is created when the enzyme, 5-monodeiodinase, found in the liver and tissue, removes single iodine from the tyrosine-iodine compound to create **T3**.

Tyrosine is a precursor for the thyroid hormone and a deficiency in tyrosine leads to hypothyroidism.

Drugs That Interfere With Thyroid

There are certain drugs that will interfere with your thyroid function, such as lithium. Other drugs that also interfere are,

Amiodarone – a heartbeat regulating drug
Colchicine – used to treat gout
Fluoxetine - used to treat depression or obsessive-compulsive disorder

Interferon-alfa - used to treat certain types of leukemias, lymphomas, or skin melanomas

Potassium iodine - Potassium iodide protects the thyroid against internal uptake of radioiodines due nuclear reactor accident

As you can see, there are a variety of drugs that affect your thyroid. If you are on any type of drug, do you know how this drug is affecting your thyroid function? If you are on drugs, try to find out how you can reduce the use of these drugs, by finding natural remedies that do the same thing as these drugs.

Other Risk Factors

If you smoke, lack folate, lack vitamin B12, have pernicious anemia or have high levels of homocysteine, these conditions been associated with hypothyroidism. Excess homocysteine comes from eating too much meat and lacking vitamin B12, B6, and Folic Acid.

Hypothyroidism

When your thyroid is not putting out enough T3 and T4, you will have hypothyroidism. This causes all your body functions, including your brain, start to slow down. You are no longer the active, smart, or persistent person you were before. You can reverse this condition and bring your thyroid function back to normal.

Hyperthyroidism

If you thyroid is putting out too much T3 and T4, you will have hyperthyroidism. This condition will cause your body to speed up in many different ways. You will be nervous, lose weight, and have a fast heartbeat.

Fixing Your Thyroid

Fixing or bringing your thyroid back to health is not just a process where only your thyroid is targeted with foods and natural remedies. If you have a slow or fast working thyroid, then your whole body needs attention.

Your thyroid is not an independent organ in your body, but works together with all other body parts. If your thyroid is not functioning right, than other parts of your body are affected and have been reduced in function.

Here is what you need to do to get your thyroid fixed.

Cleanse your body
Test your thyroid function
Eat using the body cycles
Eat for an alkaline body
Drink special juices and tonics
Take supplements and remedies
Exercise to strengthen your thyroid

Calcitonin

One other important hormone that the thyroid releases is called calcitonin. This hormone controls your calcium blood level. When you are low in blood calcium, calcitonin activates the release of calcium from your bones. This is important to know. If your thyroid is not working right, this affects your blood calcium balance and leads to calcium and bone related issues.

3: Drugs Used For Thyroid Conditions

There are many pharmaceutical drugs that are frequently prescribed by doctors for thyroid conditions. In addition there is also a natural medications that is recommended by alternative medical practitioners.

One of the most popular drugs used by doctors is Synthroid. Other drugs used are unithroid, levoxyl, and cytomel – liothyronine.

Synthroid or Levothyroxine - Synthetic T4

Synthroid is used for thyroid hormone replacement and for hypothyroidism and provides a synthetic T4. This drug Levothyroxine or Synthroid is the most common drug prescribed by doctors. The other brands like Levoxyl, Levothroid, and Unithroid also provide the synthetic T4. These other brands are simply made with different filler material.

Liothyronine - Synthetic T3

Levothyroxine and Cytomel are often used together to treat hypothyroidism. These two drugs provide a synthetic **T3.** If your body is not able to convert the T4 into T3, the use of these two drugs helps to overcome this inability.

Thyrolar (Liotrix) - Synthetic T3 and T4

Thyrolar or the drug Liotrix is a synthetic T3 and T4 combination. This drug is not used by most doctors, but when they want to provide you with both T3 and T4 they will use this drug.

Generic Thyroid Drugs

Here is a list of the generic thyroid drugs.
Levothyroxine
L-thyroxine
Liothyronine
Liotrix
Methimazole
Propylthiouracil
PTU
Natural Thyroid
Thyrotropin alfa

Thyroid Drug Brands

Here is a list of thyroid drug brands.
Armour Thyroid
Cytomel
Levothroid
Levoxyl
Naturethroid
Synthroid
Tapazole
Thyrogen
Thyrolar
Unithroid
Westhroid

Armour Thyroid

Armour Thyroid is a natural thyroid, which is derived from the thyroid gland of pigs. The original product provided many people with help and relief for their thyroid issues. There are now many reports from users of this product that since 2009 when this product formulation was changed, they have had many side effects. To read many of the complaints on this product, you can go to **Armour Thyroid**.

Side Effects Of Drugs

All drugs have side effects, especially if used for a long time.

Here are some of the side effects of the thyroid drugs listed above.

headache
sleep problems (insomnia)
feeling nervous or irritable
fever, hot flashes, sweating
pounding heartbeats or fluttering in your chest
changes in your menstrual periods or
appetite changes, weight changes
Slight hair loss
allergic reaction.

4: Testing Your Thyroid

Here is a thyroid test you can do in your home. It's called the Barnes Basal Temperature Test. This test is not to be considered an absolute accurate test for determining whether you have a thyroid condition. It is a test that can suggest whether you need to go see a doctor for further thyroid tests. It is a test to see if the symptoms you have correspond to hypo or hyperthyroidism.

Here's how to do the test.

It is best to use a mercury thermometer. Unfortunately, these thermometers are now banned. So, you need to use a digital thermometer. If you do have a mercury one, then shake it down, so the mercury level is below 90 degrees F. You may also want to go to a medical supplies store and ask for a BBT thermometer to measure body temperature in a thyroid test.
Do this test, when you first wake up in the morning. Do not move much so as not to heat up your body. Grab your digital thermometer and turn it on.

Place the tip of the thermometer in the deepest crease in your underarm. Then wait for it to beep. It does not beep keep it there for 5 minutes. If you are using a glass thermometer, leave it in your underarm for 10 minutes.

Record your temperature. Do this test for 3 days in a row and compute the average body temperature.

If you have a period, do not test during the first five days of your period. Wait until the sixth day to start. All others can test any time of the month.

Here is how to interpret your results.
97.8 to 98.2 F – is consider normal thyroid function
97.6 F or below – hypothyroidism

98.3 F or above – indicates possible hyperthyroidism

If you have been diagnosis with thyroid problems, it would be a good idea to do this basal temperature test, before you start taking drugs. This would serve as your base temperature. As you take drugs, continue to monitor your temperature to see if you have any changes. This will help you determine if the drug you are using is helpful or not.

Remember, this temperature test is not absolutely perfect, so use this information with other information you have, to determine how accurate this test is.

5: Cleansing Toxic Matter from Your Thyroid

One of the first things you need to do to get started on getting a healthier Thyroid is to do a two to three day colon and blood cleanse. This is an important step because you want to remove toxins and mucus from your intestinal tract – stomach, small intestine, colon, and many other body organs and thyroid. In this three day cleanse, you will also remove toxins from within your cells and lymph liquid.

This cleanse will pullout many acids, acid wastes, and toxins you have floating around in your body. This cleansing will make your body more alkaline.

This cleanse will clean out your blood and neutralize many of the acids in your body that are causing you harm. The cleanse will also pull out excess body water and reduce any edema that you might have. This will happen because this cleanse promotes urination and bowel movements.

Constipation

Part of this cleanse is to help you have regular bowel movements. If you do not have one to two bowel movements per day, your body will become toxic. Some toxins are often converted to fat. Keeping regular helps to keep your body clear of toxins and helps to keep your weight down.

To help you clear out your colon, there are two ways to do this. You can take Oxypowder during your three day cleanse or you can drink prune juice every day.

In this cleanse, you will only be drinking vegetable juices, fruit juices and eating some fruits for three days. Doing a juice cleanse can give you some side effects, where you feel nausea or slightly sick.

Not everyone will get these effects. If you feel sick, this is a sign that you are stirring up toxins in your stomach and elsewhere in your body, and as you get rid of these toxins you will begin to feel better.

In her extensive book, Cooking For Healthy Healing, 1991, Linda Rector-page, N.D., Ph.D., talks about what a fast does, "Fasting works by self-digestion. During a cleanse, the body in its infinite wisdom, will decompose and burn only the substances and tissue that are damaged, diseased, or unneeded, such as abscesses, tumors, excess fat deposits, and congestive wastes. Even a relatively short fast can accelerate elimination from the liver, kidneys, lungs and skin, often causing dramatic changes as masses of accumulated waste is expelled. Live foods and juices can literally pick up dead matter from the body and carry it away."

So, here's what you need to do to get started.

The Day Before The Cleanse

Buy the following juices for this cleanse a few days before or the day before your cleanse.
Organic apple juice – one gallon
Organic apples – 3 for one day, 10 apples for three days
Organic prune juice – 1/2 gallon
Organic Cherry juice – 1/2 gallon
Carrots for your juicer or carrot juice – one quart

The day before the fast, eat a large salad and two apples at dinner time. This will give you plenty of fiber to scrub the walls of your colon, as you move fecal matter out of your colon the following day.

Cleansing The Colon

If you chose to use Oxy-Powder, then here is where you can

buy it on the internet: <u>Get Oxy-Powder</u>

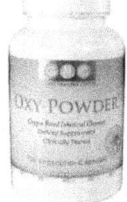 The night before you start your weight loss program, take four to five Oxy-Powder capsules. If you need to lose a lot of weight, then take five to six capsules the night before and just before you go to bed.

Now, Oxy-Powder is not a laxative so it is not addictive. What these capsules do is supply oxygen to your colon, which dissolves the hard fecal matter that has built up over time and has not wanted to come out.

Because this bottle of Oxy-Powder has 125 capsules, you can take 1 to 3 capsules during the next 30 days.

Oxy-Powder causes your stools to become watery, since it is dissolving the hard matter in your colon. Don't be concern that you have diarrhea like symptoms. Also, this three day cleanse will cause you to have watery stools, since you are on a diet of juices and fruits.

If you chose to use prune juice to clear out your colon, this procedure will be described below.

First day of colon cleanse

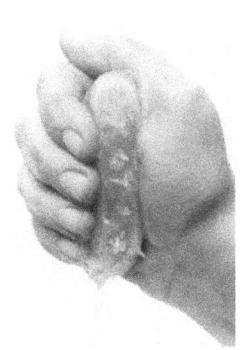 Do this cleanse on a Saturday, Sunday or any other day that you don't have to go anywhere. You may be going to the bathroom all day and at times you need to be there quick. But, you can do this cleanse even during a work day.

The first morning, you will have a bowel movement when you wake up, because of the Oxy-Powder. After that, go do your lemon drink.

Lemon Juice Drink - Every morning when you first get up, drink a glass of slightly warm water with the juice of 1/2 lemon. This will remove mucus from your intestinal tract and detoxify your liver.

Prune Juice Colon Cleanse

If you decided to use prune juice to clean out your colon, instead of Oxy-Powder, then here is what you need to do.
But you can also do prune juice, if you have done the Oxy-powder since the prune juice is filled with minerals and nutrients that will cleanse your body.

About 1/2 hour after your lemon drink, take 8 oz. of prune juice.

10 minutes later drink another 8 oz. of prune juice
10 minutes later again drink another 8 oz. of prune juice
wait 20 minutes than drink 8 oz. of apple juice
wait 30 minutes than drink another 8 oz. of apple juice

If you haven't sped to the bathroom yet, you will in a little while.

Now drink 8 oz. of apple juice every hour until the end of the day. You can stop drinking apple juice around 5pm. You can use different fruit juices or vegetable juices in place of apple juice, but, just make sure you drink mostly apple juice.

During the day and evening, you can eat 1 or 2 apples and other fruits.

Second Day Of The Colon Cleanse

During the second day, you can drink different kinds of juices and eat 2-6 apples. You can drink any kind of juice be it fruit or vegetable. A combination of fruit and vegetable juice is good. You can add other fruits to eat such as watermelon, melon, oranges, and strawberries.

Third Day of The Colon Cleanse

The third day is like the second day where you can drink different kinds of juice and eat 2-6 apples or other fruit.

On this day you can eat other fruit like mango, watermelon, cantaloupe, and pineapple. At the end of this day, you can eat a salad with a variety of vegetables.

Fourth Day Start Of Colon Cleanse

You can continue to use Oxypowder at 2 capsules every night for the rest of the month.

Now you ready to go to the next step, so let's get stated.

6: Testing Your Body for Destructive Acids

Here are 3 simple tests that you can do with your pH paper. These tests can give you an idea of how alkaline your body is and how strong your alkaline reserves are. Write down your readings and keep track of each test.

Saliva Test

Here is a simple test you can perform on your saliva that will give you an idea of where you stand with your body pH level. Your saliva contains mineral salts that keep it alkaline at 7.4. If your body is deficient in alkaline food or minerals, it will take the minerals from your saliva causing it to drop in pH.

Keep in mind there are some inaccuracies with this method, since your body fluid are always in transition. This test simply gives you an idea of what your saliva pH is at that moment. Use this information for you own education. Then as you begin to change your eating habits and life style, you can retest to see if there is a difference.

Another important issue related to pH is oxygen level. Tissue and cells have more oxygen available to them when your body pH is 7.4 as compared to when it is 6.4.

It has been found that the average American's tissue pH is between 5.5 and 6.0. This indicates that they have a severe lack of oxygen in their cells and lymph liquid. Lack of oxygen in the body is known to create serious terminal diseases. It is oxygen that destroys all types of bacteria and pathogens that live inside your body and make you ill.

Those of you with acid bodies and that lack cell and lymph oxygen can correct your condition by learning what it takes to bring your body back to an alkaline level. This will give your body a chance to repair tissue and organs, provided they have not been severely damaged.

By testing your pH regularly, you can decide the validity of using pH litmus paper to determine the level of your health. As you make changes, you can test your saliva and urine to see if the pH litmus color changes.

You need to take this test for 3 days and at least 3 times a day and get an average value so that you can establish a base line or a starting point for yourself.

Purchase some pH litmus paper at a drug store, laboratory outlet or order it through the internet. The better pH paper you can <u>buy is on Amazon</u>, with a .25 increment in pH change Gather saliva in your mouth then swallow. Do this two times. Place the pH paper under your tongue to wet it or spit on it. Let it sit for less than a minute and record the pH.

Do this test around 1 hour before eating or around 2 hours after eating.

Saliva and Lemon Test

Now, do this test immediately, after you do the saliva test above.

Squeeze half of lemon juice in one ounce of water and swish it around in your mouth for 5 seconds or so, then spit it out Wait one minute.

Now, measure your mouth's pH with litmus paper. Just place the paper into your mouth and wet it.

Now compare the color and pH value of this reading with your first pH saliva reading. This reading should have a higher alkaline reading than your first saliva reading. For example first saliva reading might be 6.3 then lemon test might be 6.8.

If this reading has a higher alkaline reading, it means you have alkaline reserves. The higher the alkaline reading you have the stronger your alkaline reserves. A small alkaline upward change means you have alkaline reserves, but they are not as strong as they should be.

If your pH reading does not change from your first reading or actually goes down by becoming more acidic, then your alkaline reserves are weak and you need to make some major changes in the way you eat. In this course, I will show you what you will need to do to bring up your alkaline reserves so that you will not be susceptible to serious diseases.

Urine pH test

There have been clinical studies indicating that urine pH is an accurate reflection of your body responding to the production acid waste.

Each time you test your urine, note what you eat in your evening meal. Eating a high evening, protein meal, which is an acid meal, will require more alkaline ash to neutralize your acid dinner, during the night. If you eat a meal high in vegetables and little protein then your body should easily neutralize your meal by morning.

Here's how to do the urine pH test

In the morning when you urinate, allow it to flow for a second and then wet your pH litmus paper with urine.

If your urine pH is below 6.4, this indicates that your body did not have enough alkaline minerals or ions to neutralize your evening dinner. In addition, you do not have enough alkaline mineral reserves to protect your body from acid damage to your cells and tissues.

Your morning urine should be between 6.7 and 7.4, indicating that your alkaline reserves are in good shape. Of course the closer you are to 7.4 the better and this is the pH you should strive for.

If your morning urine is over 7.4 and higher, this indicates your body is going into an emergency state, using ammonia from the liver in an effort to reduce your acid body. You may read as high as 8.0 indicating for sure you are producing ammonia to neutralize your acid dinner. To change this will require a substantial change in your eating habits. Sometimes you can smell that your urine is ammonia like.

Test your urine for 7 days to see if it remains consistent. Record this information to see how it changes, as you progress and change your eating habits.

If your initial pH tests indicate that you have an acid body, then depending on how acidic it is this will determine how long you have work to change your body's acid levels.

Children with an acid body will respond quickly to good changes in eating habits, whereas adults, depending on age, can see results in 5 weeks and up to a year.

7: Fruits That Help Burn Thyroid Acids

Minerals

Moving your body more toward alkalinity is what will give you the best thyroid health. When you have thyroid problems, getting more minerals in your body is the first step. An alkaline body prevents your body from becoming ill and forming deadly diseases, like joint problems, organ degradation, body pain, skin eruptions, cancer, and system weaknesses.

Removing un-necessary acids from your body will improve your immune system. The stronger your immune system is the better it is capable of keeping your thyroid and the rest of your body free of disease.

If have thyroid problems and other sicknesses, then all of the chemicals inside fruits and vegetables will help to revive your health. This is provided that your tissue damage has not gone beyond repair.

The minerals most important in changing and maintaining your body in an alkaline condition are sodium, potassium, chloride, calcium, phosphorus, magnesium, and sulfur.

Acid Binding

There are certain minerals that are called acid binding. And these are minerals, as mentioned earlier, are the most important ones in fruits, Sodium, potassium, chloride, calcium, phosphorus, magnesium, because they are acid binding.

What acid binding means is when you eat fruits with these

minerals, your cells, after metabolism, create an alkaline ash. This ash will seek out acids in your body and bind with them to neutralize them. These captured acids are routed out of your body through your urine, stools, and breathe.

Keeping Healthy

One of the most important parts of health is keeping the lymph liquid around your cells clean and free of toxins. If your body is inefficient in removing toxins from your body, it will store them in weak organs and tissue.

Thyroid cysts consist of liquid that contains toxic matter that is being stored by your body. As you become more toxic, the cyst will grow larger. If you have cysts in other parts of your body, these also grow when your body becomes more toxic.

To do this you need provide alkaline minerals to occupy the lymph liquid and you need to remove the acids that accumulate in that liquid and in all parts of your body tissue. You can do this by detoxifying your body and providing alkaline minerals for your lymph liquid.

Body Detoxification

The highest priority of the body is to detoxify itself. One of the best way to help your body detoxify is to provide minerals that bind with acids that are in the cells, tissues, organs, and muscles. What these alkaline acid binding minerals do is to pull out the toxins that are dispersed throughout your body.

With the help of the liver which detoxifies the blood, the kidney that removes impurities from the blood and the lungs which removes the CO_2 which results from alkaline acid binding, your body is constantly detoxifying itself. But when it is over loaded with acid toxins from your lifestyle, a complete detox of your body becomes impossible.

Emotional Toxins

But there is another factor that creates acid in the body and that is emotions that are occur through life stresses, like work pressures, divorce, friendship problems, martial issues, and other similar problems. These emotional problems create acidic molecules that embed themselves into your tissues just like food acids.

Body Organs

All body organs function to rid the body of acid waste or toxins. Lack of acid binding food causes deterioration of the function of these organs. Each organ has a specific function in the elimination and neutralization of acid wastes and it does this in conjunction with acid binding minerals.

Here is a list of fruits, vegetables and other foods that have the highest alkaline minerals and the highest acid production. The percentage number next to these foods indicates the strength of the alkaline minerals or the acid minerals.

The closer to 100% the more effective these foods are as an acid reducing food. However you should be eating all foods throughout the list not just the ones at the top of the list.

The percentage assigned to these fruits is based on fresh fruits and vegetables that are organic and not cooked, canned or mixed with sugar. If they are cook or otherwise processed in some fashion, this will slightly reduce their effectiveness as an acid binding. However, they will still be effective in acid binding.

Acid Binding Fruits With Alkaline Minerals

In the list below are fruits and vegetables with alkaline minerals that create acid binding salts in your body, used to neutralize acid wastes. Foods above 50% in value are more acid binding, which means they will more trap or bind with acid wastes. Foods below 50% are more acid producing and are called alkaline binding, since they tie up or bind with alkaline minerals.

To create an alkaline body, you need to eat 80% acid binding food and 20% alkaline binding food. Work towards this end and you will slowly move your body from acid to alkaline. Here is the list of foods to eat in the order of priority.

Fruits

Fruits at 100% Acid Binding – Best fruits To Eat
Lemons, melons – any type, watermelon
Fruits at 93% Acid Binding – Great fruits To Eat
Cantaloupes, dried dates, dried figs, limes, mango, and papaya
Fruits at 87% Acid Binding – Still Great Fruits To Eat
Kiwis, passion fruit, pineapples, raisins, umeboshi plums
Fruits at 80% Acid Binding – Eat These Fruits
Apricots, avocados, bananas, fresh dates, fresh figs, currants, gooseberries grapes, grapefruits guavas, kumquats, nectarines, pears, persimmons, quince, berries, cactus
Fruits at 73% Acid Binding – Still Fruits To Eat
Apples, oranges, peaches, pomegranate, raspberries, sour grapes, strawberries, carob
Fruits at 67% Acid Binding – Still Neutralizes Acids
Cherries, fresh coconut
Herbal Teas From Leaves at 73% to 86% acid binding
Alfalfa, mint, sage, spearmint, raspberry strawberry comfrey
All Herbs and Spices at 67% to 73% Acid Binding
Fruits At 40% to 47% - Eat less of these fruits
Blueberries, cranberries, plums, prunes
All Fruit Juices from a juicer 100% Acid Binding

Vegetables

Here is the list of vegetables to eat in order of priority. All of these vegetable will neutralize acid, since they contain minerals that are acid binding.

Vegetables at 93% Acid Binding – best vegetables to eat
Kelp, Seaweed, Watercress, Asparagus

Vegetables at 80% Acid Binding – Still the best to eat
Lettuce Leaf, Oyster plant, Pumpkin, Spinach, Squash, Peas, Carrots, Celery, Chard, Swiss, Dandelion greens

Vegetables at 73% Acid Binding – Great vegetables to eat
Bamboo shoots, Beets, Broccoli, Cabbage, Cauliflower, Collards, Corn, sweet, Ginger (fresh), Mushrooms, Mustard greens, Onions, Pepper, Potatoes, Green, Lima, String, Potatoes

Vegetables at 67% Acid Binding – eat plenty of these
Brussels sprouts, Cucumbers, Eggplant, Okra, Onions, Radishes, Tomatoes

Vegetable juices at 80% to 93% Acid Binding
Parsley, wheat grass, carrot, celery, etc.

Soy Bean Products at 60% Acid Binding – Limit your use of tofu since it is a genetically modified organism, GMO
Dried beans, Soy cheese, Soy milk, Tempeh, Tofu

Here are some other misc. foods to eat that are acid binding.
Starches at 80% Acid Binding
Arrowroot flour
Sugar at 73% acid Binding
Honey
Nuts and Seeds at 60 % to 67% Acid Binding
Almonds, sesame seeds, Granola, Essene Bread, Chestnuts
Misc. foods at 60% Acid Binding
Horseradish, Amaranth, Millet, Quinoa, Dried beans, Soy cheese, Soy milk,

The following foods are Alkaline binding, which means that they create acids that will bind with alkaline salts and remove them from your body. These foods when eaten in excess will create an acid body.

You should only eat around 20% of these foods in your diet and the other 80% should come from fruits and vegetables or foods that are acid binding.

NOTE: The lower the alkaline binding percentage, the more that food is acid producing.

All oils are basically at 50% and are considered neutral. This includes almond, avocado, canola, coconut, corn castor, olive, soy, sunflower oil, and etc.

Beans, starches, and nuts and seeds at 40% to 46% Alkaline Binding

Aduki, Black, Broadbean, Garbanzo, Mung, Pinto, Barley, Corn Meal, Lentils, Brans, Cashews, Coconut (dried), Pecans, Brans, Millet, Filberts, Walnuts, Pumpkin, Sunflower
Starches at 26 to 33 % Alkaline Binding
Brown Rice, Buckwheat, Oats, Spelt, Wheat Whole, Peanuts, corn, rye
Rice at 20% Alkaline Binding
White rice
Sugar at 13% Alkaline Binding
White beet or cane sugar
Meat and Fish
Meat at 26% alkaline binding
Fish With fins and scales, Shellfish - shrimp, scallops, crab lobster, oyster
Meat at 20% Alkaline Binding
Chicken, turkey, rabbit
Meat at 13% Alkaline Binding
Beef, goat, pork, lamb
Misc. Products at 13% to 26% Alkaline Binding
Liquor, wine, beer, coffee, black tea, caffeine drinks

8: Body Cycles That Help Fix Your Thyroid

Body cycles are time periods where your body is doing certain functions in your body. It does the automatically as if it was on a timer. Know what they functions are will help you get relief from your disease or to even eliminate it. You should use these cycles outline below every day.

Here are the 3 natural body cycles:

Cycle 1 time period: 4 a.m. to 12 noon

This cycle is the time where your body is eliminating toxins, acids, wastes, and derby through urine, bowel movements, and other secretions. Most people interfere with this cycle, since they are unaware of it, causing constipation, increase weight and various detrimental illnesses.

Cycle 2 time period: 12 noon to 8 p.m.

This is the time when your body should be taking in food and digesting it. By eating the right kind of food, you help your digestive process in your stomach and small intestine. This is your first and second meal of the day – lunch and dinner.

Cycle 3 time period: 8 p.m. to 4 a.m.

This is the time your body is absorbing and using food you have eaten from 12 noon to 8 p.m. Various organs are detoxifying and producing waste and moving it into your kidney and colon. When you wake up, this is the waste you should be getting rid during body cycle one.

The First Body Cycle

During the elimination cycle, 4 a.m. to 12 noon, eat and drink only green drinks, fruits and their juices or drink vegetable juices. For breakfast, eat a bowl of fruit or have a fruit smoothie made with apple juice, banana, and fruits in season. Before noontime, eat fruits as snacks. Forty-five minutes before noon eat your last fruit. You can eat and drink all the fruits and juices you want up to noontime.

Green Juices

Here are some green drinks to take. You don't have to do all of them just choose one that appeals to and do that one and rotate to the others during the month.

A green drink can help you control sugar blood levels through the production of insulin. It does this by rebuilding the pancreas so that glucagon and insulin are created throughout the day.

A green drink can be used every day. Try to use a green drink at least twice a week.

Chlorophyll

Using liquid chlorophyll is great, if you don't have a green drink.

1 – 2 oz. of liquid chlorophyll
6 oz. of distilled water
The juice of 1/2 lemon or lime

This can be drunk every day first thing in the morning.

Aside from breakfast fruits, green drinks are also a great way to start your morning. These drinks can be taken first before your fruits.

Drink one glass of water with half the juice of one lemon.

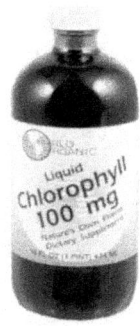

30 minutes later drink a green drink in one of two ways. You can put 1 to 2 tablespoons of liquid chlorophyll in 8 oz. of water or a capful of your favorite green powder in 8 oz. of water.

For the <u>chlorophyll drink</u>, add the juice of 1/2 lemon juice to give it some flavor. For the <u>green power</u> drinks add some honey so it is easier to drink.

Blue Green Manna

Blue Green Manna is another powder you can use. It is high in chlorophyll and enzymes in the chlorophyll. This Manna is great for regulating the pancreas. You can check out this site for capsule.

Blue Green Manna – 1 tablespoon
6 oz. of distilled water
2 oz. of pineapple, apple, or grape juice
You can add a couple of ounces of fresh pineapple, apple, and grape juice to make it more palatable. Adding a pinch of honey is another way to take a green drink.

For kids you can add the green drink or green manna into jello.

Kale and Collard Juices

Kale is very high in alkaline minerals like calcium and in vitamin A. You can mix kale juice with carrot or pineapple juice. Drinking kale or collard juices will help you absorb more calcium that you do, when you drink milk.

Mustard Greens Juice Recipe

Pure mustard greens juice has an irritating effect to the gastrointestinal tract and to the kidney. By combining the juice of mustard greens with carrot, spinach and turnip juice, you will get the strong alkaline minerals to eliminate acids.

Mustard greens have a high level of oxalic acid and should never be eaten cooked. When cooked, the oxalic acid becomes an acid that forms kidney stones.

Spinach

Here is another green drink with spinach, which can help you detoxify your body.

Spinach 2oz.
Carrot 6 oz.
Celery a small amount of this juice
Cucumber a small amount of this juice

Spinach is also high in organic oxalic acid and should not be eaten cooked. Eat it raw or juiced to get the natural oxalic acid that your body needs.

Fruit Breakfast

Fruits contain the right balance of nutrients with about 70% distilled water. Eat them without cooking them. They are easy to digest and absorb and do not stress your colon. They activate peristaltic action in your colon and help you have a bowel movement.

Use the Acid Binding Fruits listed in the previous chapter. Here are some more fruits to eat:

Apples
Apricots
Avocados
Bananas
Blueberries
Boysenberries
Cantaloupes
Cherries
Figs and dates
Grapes

Grapes
Lemons
Nectarines
Oranges
Papayas
Peaches
Pears
Persimmons
Plums
Prunes
Raspberries
Strawberries
Watermelons

Eat all melons together and not with other fruit and wait 1/2 hour before eating other fruit. Melons require specific enzymes to be digested in the stomach, so other fruit eaten with melons will just sit in your stomach, waiting to be digested and can cause gas and an acid stomach.

Fruit Pudding

Next mix a fruit pudding to take to work for a snack. Here are two different things you can do with a blender. Take these blended fruits to work in a thermos to eat when you get there.

Put into a blender

Two small or one large banana
One mango
Pineapple
One apple
1/4 of a papaya (if available)
Small amount of apple juice to make this blend into a pudding

Blend all of this for 1 – 2 minutes.

You can add lecithin granules or powdered vitamin C to make it more a tart and to preserve it.

By eating fruits during body cycle 1, you are assisting your body's elimination cycle. Fruits and juices help your body to urinate, or have a bowel movement, and eliminate toxins and acids from your body and blood. It is these toxins and acids that make you, overweight, constipated, and sick.

Eating solid food for breakfast – eggs potatoes, rice, meat, cereal, milk, and so on, the typical breakfast, interferes with your body's elimination cycle and eventually leads to sickness and excess weight.

It takes over 3 hours to digest heavy and solid food. The food you should be eating in the morning should digest quickly. This helps you to activate peristaltic colon action to create a bowel movement and to continue your body's detoxification and elimination process.

Heavy food slows down the elimination of toxins from your body and this causes chime and toxins to remain in your colon longer than necessary. These toxins then get stored in your body as fat and acids.

It takes 1 to 1 1/2 hour or so to digest fruits and fruit juices. Because of this, they help to cleanse your body of waste during the time from 4am to noontime.

So, if you are not already having fruit and fruit and vegetables juices for breakfast and snacks, start slowing changing your eating habits, if you want to lose weight and feel better.

The Second Natural Body Cycle

Here is the second body cycle and it occurs from 12 noon to 8 p.m.

This is the time when your body should be taking in food and digesting it. During this period, it is time to eat solid food. What you eat has to be in alignment with what your stomach can do.

Here's how your stomach works. Generally, it can only digest one solid food at a time.

A solid food is one that does not contain 70% water, like fruits and vegetables do, and whose water has been eliminated by heat or other food processes, in other words cooked.

Your stomach can only work on one solid food at a time, so your lunch and dinner should only have one solid food. A lunch can consist of chicken and a green salad, fish and a green salad, tuna and a green salad, shrimp and a green salad, beef and a green salad.

Mixing a protein meal with carbohydrates is giving the stomach two solid foods at the same time, which require different concentrations of digestive juices.

When you eat any animal protein, avoid eating it with nonstarchy vegetables - artichokes, yams, sweet potatoes, carrots, oats, peas, potatoes, rice, wheat, winter squash and corn. These vegetables breakdown into sugars that coat your protein food and this causes a chemical process called glycation, which creates inflammation and lowers your immunity. In addition, this combination of protein and starches are difficult to digest and disrupt your second body cycle

When you eat animal protein, eat it with broccoli, cabbage, cauliflower, celery, cucumber, garlic, green beans, leafy greens onions, garlic, wakame, dulse, and zucchini.

Giving the stomach more than it can handle interrupts the elimination cycle 1 and reduces the energy that you need for the elimination cycle.

Here's how you can help your body's cycle 2 to be more effective.

Eat only one solid food with vegetables during lunch or dinner.

Lunch can be one meat or seafood with a fresh vegetable salad that is nonstarchy.

Or you can eat only brown or red rice or other grains, with both starchy and nonstarchy vegetables, with no meat.

Limit the amount of water you drink during meals. Excess water will dilute your digestive acids and slow down digestion of your food.

Avoid drinking sodas, tea or other drinks during your meals. If you need to clear your dry throat, use room temperature water. Cold liquids will slow down your digestive processes.

Eating meals with more than one solid food such as meat and potatoes, chicken and rice, fish and rice, chicken and noodles, eggs and toast, cheese and bread will diminish the energy you need during the elimination cycle

It is permissible to eat beef and chicken at the same time but not chicken and eggs or beef and nuts or chicken and beans. Eat the same type of protein at the same time, but do not mix different proteins.

It's ok to eat different types of carbohydrates at the same time, with a salad, but not with protein, since carbohydrates digest easier than protein.

Eating a variety of food at the same time leads to undigested food. Food that is partially undigested becomes acidic, which affects the health of your colon and causes constipation. When these acids are absorbed into your body, they are converted into fat and stored as toxins your body.

Eating the right combination of foods at meal time, helps you to preserve your energy for the elimination cycle and prevents you from creating spoiled food in your stomach that is converted to acid waste. It is this acid waste that results in illness and fat. This is the reason most people as they age come down with various illnesses that terminate their life early or gain excessive weight.

The Third Body Cycle

The third body cycle is the assimilation cycle and is from 8pm to 4am. This is the time the food you have eaten during the day is assimilated, absorbed and distributed throughout your body through your blood. It is the time where digested food moves into the colon as chime and is stored there for elimination. And, you should be eliminating this chime or fecal matter, when you wake up or during the morning to 12 noon.

Food eaten during the second cycle, 12 noon to 8 p.m. and that were combined and eaten properly will digest within 3 to 4 hours, whereas food not combine properly, a meal consisting of protein and carbohydrates will take up to 8 hours to pass through your stomach. During this time, your food will putrefy and ferment and become acidic. Under these conditions, you will not get many nutrients from that meal.

So, eat your last meal by 6-7 pm, so that your food digests in your stomach by the time you go to bed. After three hours later, your food will have moved into your small intestine where it is ready for assimilation.

When you go to bed 3 hours after your last meal, the next 6 hours, until 4am, your body will be absorbing the food you have eaten the previous day and moving waste into your colon.

9: Foods That Help Repair Your Thyroid

In the previous chapters, you were introduced to various concepts that you need to use to create better health. In this process of creating better health, you improve your immune system, get rid of excess body acids, create a daily detoxifying process, and strengthen your thyroid.

Now it is time to add foods that specifically target your thyroid. By eating and drinking these foods, you will strengthen and detoxifying your thyroid. Your concentration should be on these foods, but this does not mean you ignore other foods listed in the other chapters to get rid of acid and to start your morning.

Goitrongen

There are foods that have been identified as "goitrogens," which prevent iodine from being used in the thyroid. These foods are:

Sweet potato
Cabbage
Cauliflower
Turnips
Rutabaga
Canola Oil
Cassava
Pine Nuts
Mustard
Millet
Soybeans
Peanuts

However, if you cook these foods then the goitrogenic property is disabled.

Beta Caroten

First, your diet must be rich in beta carotene. Beta carotene, a carotenoid, is an antioxidant and is the yellow, orange, or red color in plants, fruits, and vegetables. When you eat food that is rich in carotene, your body converts it to vitamin A.

So why not take vitamin A supplements? Yes, you can take vitamin A supplements, but you must not take an excess of vitamin A, since it is toxic. When you eat beta carotene food, your body only converts the amount of beta carotene to vitamin A that it needs.

Also, when you eat carotene foods, they are packed with vitamins, minerals, antioxidants, and other nutrients that are balanced with the right amount of beta carotene that your body needs.

Beta Carotene powers up your immune system and protects your thyroid cells from free radical damage. Studies have shown that beta carotene reduces your risk of developing cancer.

Use the following foods in your recipes for breakfast, lunch, dinner, or snacks. They can be in the form of fresh salads, puddings, juices, or smoothies.

Spices

Spices are high in beta carotene. Because they are dried, the beta carotene is more concentrated. Use these spices in your cooking. These spices are listed in the order of highest carotene concentration.
Paprika
Cayenne pepper
Chili powders
Marjoram
Sage
Coriander

Parsley
Oregano
Cumin
Curry powder
Fresh basil
Fresh thyme

Sweet potatoes, boiled

Sweet potatoes are one of the highest foods in beta carotene. These can be used as snacks or puddings, or smoothies.

Go here for **pudding recipes**, but go easy on the sugar.
It is best to boil sweet potatoes instead of baking them. Once boiled, you can mix them slightly with other milks, such as rice dream or almond milk.

Carrots

Carrots are king of vegetables, because you can juice them and combine them with many other green vegetable juices to make them more palatable. Carrots are the vegetable you should be eating daily. Eat them both slightly cooked and raw, but cooked gives you more nutrition than raw.

Red bell peppers

Use the different color bell peppers and other chili peppers in your soup to get a high level of beta carotene. You can also use bell peppers in your salad. Use Tabasco sauce on your breakfast eggs or on other dishes you like.

Tomato Powder

If you can find tomato powder, add it to your soups.

Greens

These are the greens to concentration on. You can use them in salad, soups, or juices. When you juice them add 1/2 to 3/4 carrot juice. You can experiment with the amount of carrot juice your use. You may want to add a little bit of apple juice to sweeten the taste.

Dandelion leaves, Kale, Spinach, turnip greens, mustard greens, and collards.

Lettuces to use in your salads are the dark green and red lettuces. The more orange and red color they have the better. Other vegetables to eat are asparagus, broccoli, and Chinese cabbage.

Pumpkin and Squash

Most people know how to use pumpkin. Pumpkin and squash can be used in soups.

Fruits
The fruits that have the highest beta carotene are as follows.
Dried apricots
Raw apricots
Dried peaches
Raw red cherries
Grapefruit
Mango
Plums
Plantains
Raw guavas

There are some drugs that interfere with the absorption of beta carotene. And sometimes beta carotene will interfere with the effectiveness of a drug.

Statins – if you are taking statins, beta carotene can interfere with the effectiveness of Zocor and niacin.

Cholesterol lowering drugs – like cholestyramine and colestipol can decrease the blood levels of beta carotene by up to 40%

Weight control supplements – like Orlistat, Xenical, and Alli can decrease the absorption of beta carotene by up to 30%.

Vitamin C

The next thing you need to concentration on is getting more vitamin C into your body. Many of the foods high in beta carotene are also high in vitamin C, so this makes it easy to get more vitamin C, when you concentration on beta carotene foods.

Here are the foods high in vitamin C.

Combine the juice these three fruits – orange, grapefruit, and lemon. Use a hand juices to prepare a fresh citrus juice drink. Take one fruit of each and juice it. You can drink this first thing in the morning.

10: Tonic & Drinks That Support Your Thyroid

Thyroid Tonics

Here is a tonic for hypothyroidism. It will normalize your thyroid function. Drink this juice 3 times a day.

1/2 cup unsweetened gelatin powder
2 tablespoons brewer's yeast
1/2 to 1 cup freshly squeezed orange juice

To improve the effectiveness of this tonic, eliminate the use of sugar in soft drinks and foods. When you do this, you maximize the power of this tonic.

Mineral Tonics

Mix and drink this tonic every day.
One part carrot juice
One part celery juice
One part radish juice
2 tbs. of onion juice

Raisin Apricot Mineral Tonic

1/2 cup of raisin juice
1/2 cup of apricot juice
1 tbs. of lemon juice

Drink this tonic twice a day. You can create raisin and apricot juice by soaking their dried fruit over night with about 3/4 cup of water. In the morning, pour all the water and soaked fruit into a blender to create a pudding or smoothie.

Potassium Mineral tonic

Here is another powerful mineral tonic that will provide nutrients for your whole body. It is a tonic packed with potassium and other minerals and vitamins.
Boil distilled water and turn off heat
In a bowl put any of the following dried fruits together – peaches, apricots, raisins, prunes, and pears.
Pour hot water into the bowl and cover
Let bowl with fruits sit over night
In the morning drink one cup of this juice
Eat fruit as a breakfast

You can also take the liquid and fruit and put it into a blender. Add a bit of honey and a little bit of apple juice and blend. You can blend to make a pudding or a shake.

This tonic will help make you regular, neutralize body acid, activate kidney and detoxify body, provide iron for blood creating hemoglobin, and provide B vitamins.

Juice mineral Tonic

This tonic will provide your skin, nails, and cells with the nutrients it needs to be healthy.

Mix together the following in equal portions.
Cranberry, pineapple, berry juice and then add a tbs. of lemon juice.

Mix green tea and ginger

A tea of ginger – improves blood circulation
A cup of green tea – helps to detoxify your body and is good for your cardiovascular system.

11: Supplements That Enhance Thyroid Function

Iodine

Iodine is essential for the health of your thyroid. As mentioned earlier,

"Thyroglobulin is a protein that is created in your thyroid. When thyroglobulin and iodine combine, the thyroid hormone is created."

It is also important to note that a deficiency in selenium increases the effects of iodine deficiency. Selenium is necessary in creating a selenium enzyme, iodothyronine deiodinases, which is required for the conversion of T4 to T3. Deficiencies in vitamin A and iron can also magnify the effects of iodine deficiency.

So without iodine and selenium you are not able to create the thyroid hormones you need to maintain life. However, there are some people that are sensitive to iodine and over dose on it. The result is they develop hyperthyroidism with symptoms of nervousness, heart palpitations, sleeplessness, irritability or enlarged thyroid.

So what is the best way to get iodine into your diet? Using iodized salt is one way to get more iodine, but using a lot of salt in your diet is not healthy and some people need to minimize their use of table salt. There are also many other foods that are high in salt and should be avoided. Here are some other high sources of iodine to add to your diet.

Seaweeds

Seaweeds have the highest iodine content over all foods. It is something you need to incorporate into your diet. But you want to be careful not to overdose with it, since it can cause hyperthyroidism. Just start to use it in your diet slowly by adding seaweeds to your soups or salads. Here is a list of different sea weeds.

Icelandic kelp
Norwegian kelp
Atlantic kelp
Pacific kelps
Fucus spp
Wakame
Sargassum
Nori
Iris moss

Eating Seaweed

In many Asian countries, seaweed is soaked from 10 to 30 minutes before they use it in their miso or other cooking. This process removes around 60% of the iodine. After soaking the seaweed is thrown away.

RDA Iodine Daily Recommendations

Children 1 to 8 years... 90 mcg
Children 9 to 18 years... 120 to 150 mcg
Adults 19 years and older 150 mcg
Women pregnant ... 220 mcg
Women breast-feedng ... 290 mcg

Here are some foods that contain iodine that you can incorporate into your diet.

Seaweed, 1/4 ounce, dried... 4,500 mcg
Cod, 3 ounces... 99 mcg
Iodized salt, .035 ounce... 77 mcg
Potato with peel, baked... 60 mcg
Milk, cow, 1 cup...56 mcg
Shrimp or fish sticks... 35 mcg

Turkey breast, 3 ounces... 34 mcg
Navy beans, 1/2 cup...32 mcg
Tuna in oil, 3 ounces... 17 mcg

The adult RDA for iodine is 100-150 mcg and you can get this by eating 0.14 ounces of dried seaweeds.

However, the Food and Nutrition Board (FNB) of the Institute of Medicine has recommend 1,100 mcg/day of iodine for adults. And for children it has been set at,

Children 1-3... 200 mcg
Children 4-8... 300 mcg
Children 9-13... 600 mcg
Adolescents 14-18... 900 mcg
Adults 19 and older... 1100 mcg/day.

Iodine Toxicity

Acute iodine toxicity is quite rare and will only occur if you consume grams of iodine. In a typical natural food diet you may be consuming 2,000 mcg of iodine daily, but less than 1000 mcg is more typical.

It appears from studies made on the use of iodine that iodine supplementation is not necessary, since a good diet will provide the iodine necessary for good thyroid function.

If you have symptoms of hypothyroidism, then you might want to increase your intake of iodine high foods.

If you have the autoimmune thyroid disease like Hashimoto's thyroiditis or Graves' disease, you should **avoid** taking iodine supplements, since these diseases are not cause by the lack of iodine. In some cases, iodine may irritate these conditions.

Required Supplements

Here are the supplements that are necessary to maintain

thyroid health. If you are short on these vitamins and minerals they will affect the function of your thyroid. Make sure you supplement with them.

Selenium

It is critical that you have a daily dose of selenium. You can get it from your food or through a supplement. Selenium helps to improve your thyroid feedback system and at the same time improve the conversion of T4 to T3. It also helps in the detoxification of your body.

DHEA

Dehydroepiandrosterone, DHEA is a hormone enhancer and helps to enhance your body's metabolism.

Vitamins

Here are the vitamins that you need to have for best thyroid function.

Vitamin A, B complex, C, E, and Co Q10
You can buy the B100 complex and a good vitamin supplement.

Minerals You Need

The minerals that you need are magnesium, manganese, selenium, zinc, copper, molybdenum.

Lack of these minerals will prevent the conversion of T4 to T3.

Special Thyroid Formulations

Here is a product that has all the minerals and tyrosine that you need, with a thyroid glandular, so check it out. Makes it easy to get the nutrients you need to get started right away with your thyroid issues.

Enzymatic Therapy - Metabolic Advantage

Here is another thyroid formulation. It doesn't have the minerals, but has a variety of herbs that can provide the minerals you need. Usually herbs work on the whole body, so you may prefer this product. Here are the ingredients for this product:

Gaia Herbs Thyroid Support

L-Tyrosine   300 mg
Coleus Forskholii root (Coleus forskholii)   154 mg
Ashwagandha root (Withania somnifera)   120 mg
Schizandra berry (Schizandra chinensis)   78 mg
Kelp fronds (Laminaria digitata)   65 mg
Bladderwrack fronds (Fucus vesiculosis)   28 mg

Daily Supplement Requirement

Here is the daily dose of the various nutrients you need. So if you want to buy them separately, you can.

Iodine – 1mg
Selenium – 200 to 600 mcg or ug
Zinc – 10 mg
Tyrosine – 500 – 1000 mg
Melatonin – 1 – 6 mg
DHEA – 25 mg
Co Q10 – 100-200 mg

Just remember that the food you eat will also be providing you with the above nutrients, but it's always best to supplement when you are trying to fix a health issue. The body will use what it needs and get rid of what it doesn't, provided you don't overdose.

12: Exercises That Strengthen Your Thyroid

Caution: If you have not exercised for a while, take this program slowly and work into it. If you feel some concern about exercising and your health make sure you see your doctor.

As I have mentioned, you need a good cardiovascular system to your overall health. The slow degradation of your cardiovascular system is reflected in all aspects of your wellbeing.

So let's get started with the exercises you need to do. You will be doing these exercises in a different way than you are used to. Most exercise gurus tell you that you need aerobics to strengthen your hearts. Exercise studies have shown that this is not the way to strengthen your heart; in fact it does the opposite. When you go to the gym for and do repetitive exercises for over 20 minutes you are not strengthening your heart or are you going to lose weight that will stay off.

In his e-book called Pace, Dr. Al Sears, outline a new way of exercising to strengthen your cardiovascular system. He says that,

"During twenty years of working with extremely fit athletes, patients with diseased or injured hearts and average people in between, one thing is apparent: Doing what we have come to accept as 'cardio' exercise is a waste of your time and effort.
It doesn't build what your heart really needs. It doesn't increase your heart's ability to respond to the real demands. In fact, for all your effort, you only reduce your ability to handle suddenly demanding events that may come your way – the last thing you want."

During the short, fast exercises from 2 to 15 minutes, you are burning calories supplied by:

The first couple of minutes the energy comes from your ATP – cell energy.

After 2 minutes the energy comes from the carbohydrates stored in your muscle tissue.

After 15-20 minutes the energy starts to come from stored fat When you exercise is at a moderate rate, you are burning 40% carbohydrates and 55% fat. When you exercise at a high intensity, you are burning 95% carbohydrates and 3% fat. You want to exercise in a way and for time duration where you are burning carbohydrates and very little fat.

When you exercise and burn fat, you are telling your body that you need fat when you exercise. So when you come to exercise next time, your body will have stored fat to sustain the energy you need during exercising. Your body is storing and building up your fat reservoirs each time you eat so it can sustain the moderate intensity exercises that you do.

One other thing, when you are just at your rest state, not exercising, you are burning 35% carbohydrates and 65% fat. What this means is that you will continue to store fat if you do not exercise at all. You are telling your body that when you do nothing, you need fat to be able to do nothing. So when you eat, your body will store fat from the food you eat. No exercise is a destructive activity for your body.

If you practice high intensity exercise your chance of a heart disease is 100% less than those who do aerobic exercise.

Anaerobic Exercise

The way you will exercise is to exercise for short duration at high intensity. This is called anaerobic exercise. To do anaerobic exercise, you exercise at a pace you can't sustain for more than a short time. You will be breathing hard and are asking your lungs for more oxygen than they can give you. Because of this, your lungs need to expand to get more oxygen. You are now building your lungs for greater capacity. You are now burning more carbohydrates than fat. And, in the time between exercising your fat is burned, since your body determines it is not necessary to keep fat for energy, since carbohydrates are what is really needed.

Exercising

As you do Pace exercising, you will change your routine each time you exercise. Instead of exercising longer, you will increase the exercise intensity and the resistive element of exercising.

To start this exercise program, start with a 10 minute workout. You can do your exercise on a stair-stepper, stationary bike, treadmill, run, swim, or ride your bike. You will want to check with your doctor, if you:

Have had not a medical checkup during the past two years
Are over 50

Are 26 lbs or over
Have heart pains, chest pains, or rapid heart palpitations after you exercise
Are taking heart medication or have a pace maker
Have angina, heart murmur or any type of heart disease
Have a relative that died of a heart attack before age 60
Have a hard time breathing and have any type of respiratory disease – asthma, emphysema.

Monitoring Your Heart Rate

To check your progress in your exercise program, you need to check your:

Resting heart rate

Maximum heart rate for your age
Maximum heart rate during exercise
Recovery heart rate

Resting Heart Rate

Your resting heart rate is before you exercise. The lower your resting heart rate is the healthier you are, unless you have a pacemaker or have heart problems. Normal rate is 60 to 100 pulses per minute. If you are really in good shape then your pulse will be 40 – 60 per minute

To determine your resting heart rate, get a second timer and count the number of pulses you have in 10 seconds. Then multiple this number by 6 to get your pulse rate per minute. To get a more accurate reading of your pulse rate do you 10 second reading 3 time and get an average of these readings.

Maximum Heart Rate for Your Age

The maximum heart rate for your age is that heart rate that you should strive for during your exercise to get the best benefit of your exercise. You calculate this rate by subtracting your age from 220. During your exercise, you want to achieve 60- 80 % of your maximum heart rate for your age. Here is a sample chart you can use to see different heart rates for your heart:

Age	Max Pulse 220-age	60% of max pulse	80% of max pulse
35	185	111	148
40	180	108	144
45	175	105	140
50	170	102	136
55	165	99	132
60	160	96	128
65	155	93	124
70	150	90	120

Based on your physical condition, use these numbers as guide lines.

Maximum Heart Rate During Exercise

The maximum heart rate is the highest rate your pulse achieved during your exercise. Use the chart above to evaluate where you are, with respect to the heart rate for your age.

During exercise, if your heart rate is on the lower end of the heart rate for your age, you will want to exercise harder to get your heart rate up. If you are really out of shape, then take it easy and work up to the 60% and eventually to the 80% heart rate, as you improve your stamina.

You can measure your exercise heart rate the same way you calculate your resting heart rate.

Recovery Heart Rate

The heart recovery rate is the time it takes for your maximum heart rate to recover to your resting heart rate. As you exercise more, the less time will be required for you to achieve your heart recovery rate. When you exercise for your chosen time, clock your recovery rate, since a change in this rate indicates you are improving in your healthy.

You will see change in this rate in one month. Do not do your next exercise until you reach your resting heart rate. So you will be cycling from resting rate –exercise rate – resting rate – exercise rate – resting rate. Do ten of these cycles as an exercise routine.

Caution: See your doctor before you start an exercise program or if the following conditions occur:

Your heart rate, after maximum exercise, does not come down within a few minutes
You feel dizzy or faint

You have chest pains or are short of breath
You have rapid heartbeat or irregular heartbeat

This is exercise program is the basic outline of Dr. Sears' PACE program. His e-book takes off to higher levels of exercise methods, so if you want to see his full program you can buy his e-book called Pace.

13: A Program to Fix Your Thyroid

A lot of material has been covered and you may not know where to start or what to do first. Here is an outline of one way you can start. This program is flexible, so you can decide what you want to do first. The idea is to make a list of the direction you want to go in and get all the items and materials in place to make it happen.

Thyroid Test

Do a thyroid temperature test. This gives you a base line so that as you make changes to your eating habits, you can see if it is affecting your thyroid. You will need a digital thermometer.

Test Your body's pH

Next, you want to do a pH test as outline in a previous chapter. This also serves as a pH base line. You want to see if you body's acid is reduced and by how much. You main goal is to try to make your body's pH between 7.0 and 7.4. When you get there, you know that your body is alkaline and now you need to maintain this condition. You will need to buy pH litmus paper.

Body Cleanse

You can do a one, two or three day body cleanse. This will help you get rid of some toxins that might be affecting your thyroid. If you can do a longer time, that is even better. You can try a three day cleanse.

Body Cycles

Revisit the idea of the body cycles, especially the first body cycle. First thing each morning, drink lemon water, lemon chlorophyll, or a citrus combination drink. Follow this with a green drink of your choice.

Breakfast Acid Binding

After about 1 hour or so mix a pudding or shake using the fruits that are the best for acid binding.

Fruits at 100% Acid Binding - Lemons, melons – any type, watermelon

Fruits at 93% Acid Binding - Cantaloupes, dried dates, dried figs, limes, mango, papaya

Fruits at 87% Acid Binding –Kiwis, passion fruit, pineapples, raisins, umeboshi plums

Fruits at 80% Acid Binding –Apricots, avocados, bananas, fresh dates, fresh figs, currants, gooseberries grapes, grapefruits guavas, kumquats, nectarines, pears, persimmons, quince, berries, cactus

Fruits at 73% Acid Binding – Apples, oranges, peaches, pomegranate, raspberries, sour grapes, strawberries, carob

You can eat these fruits as a bowl of fruits each morning and take some of these fruits for morning or afternoon snacks.
You can also prepare and drink vegetable juices in the morning.

Cycle 2 and 3 – Lunch and Dinner

During lunch and dinner, you want to eat those vegetable in a salad or cooked that are the highest in acid binding. Just make sure you eat every day some raw vegetables.

Acid Binding Vegetables

Vegetables at 93% Acid Binding – Kelp, Seaweed, Watercress, Asparagus

Vegetables at 80% Acid Binding – Lettuce Leaf, Oyster plant, Pumpkin, Spinach, Squash, Peas, Carrots, Celery, Chard, Swiss, Dandelion greens

Vegetables at 73% Acid Binding – Bamboo shoots, Beets, Broccoli, Cabbage, Cauliflower, Collards, Corn, sweet, Ginger (fresh), Mushrooms, Mustard greens, Onions, Pepper, Potatoes, Green, Lima, String, Potatoes

Spices With High Beta Carotene

You should also incorporate those foods that are high in beta carotene. Use these spices in your cooking,

Paprika
Cayenne pepper
Chili powders
Marjoram
Sage
Coriander
Parsley
Oregano
Cumin
Curry powder
Fresh basil
Fresh thyme
Lunch, Dinner, Or Snack Foods High In Beta Carotene

Sweet potatoes, boiled

Sweet potatoes boiled are one of the highest foods in beta carotene. Eat these 3 times a week for a couple of weeks. Then eat them once a week.

Carrots

Carrots are king of vegetables. Eat them raw, cooked or in juices.

Red bell peppers

Use the different color bell peppers and other chili peppers in your soup to get a high level of beta carotene.

Tomato Powder

If you can find tomato powder, add it to your soups.

Greens

You can use greens in salad, soups, or juices. When you juice them add 1/2 to 3/4 cup carrot juice to 1/4 or more of green juice.

Dandelion leaves, Kale, Spinach, turnip greens, mustard greens, and collards.

Lettuces to use in your salads are the dark green and red lettuces. The more orange and red color they have the better.

Important Vegetables

Other important vegetables to eat for selenium
Asparagus
Broccoli
Chinese cabbage
Garlic
Mushroom

Pumpkin and Squash

Most people know how to use pumpkin. Pumpkin and squash can be used in soups.

Fruits

The fruits that have the highest beta carotene are as follows:

Dried apricots
Raw apricots
Dried peaches
Raw red cherries
Grapefruit
Mango
Plums
Plantains
Raw guavas

Supplements

Go back to the supplements that you should be taking, and take them with meals.

Take a thyroid formulation to supplement you're eating program. Also add some of the vitamins recommended.

Make sure you supplement with selenium and zinc.

Exercise

Start exercising so that you can help detoxify your body. Exercising of any kind helps to circulate your lymph liquid to help detoxify it.

There you have it a detailed program that you can vary according your preference. Do something every week and don't try to do all of this in the first week. Work into the program slowly, so that it will become part of what you do.

14: Author and Resources

Rudy Silva is a natural consultant nutritionist educated in the United State in Nutrition and Physics. He is a graduate from the San Jose State University in California. He is author of 30 other e-books on natural remedies. He has authored a newsletter in natural remedies for over 4 years. He has many websites promoting special recommended products and information.

Resource page

Here are some of the other kindle e-books about natural remedies that have been written by this author. You can see the entire list at:

http://tinyurl.com/b2f7wd3

Constipation Remedies
Best Constipated Women Natural Cures

Essential Fatty Acids
Taking The Mystery Out Of Essential Fatty acids
Amazing Fish Oil Benefits Revealed

Nutrition Remedies
Fast Healing Juice Nutrition Therapy: Nutrition Tips 3
Magnesium Nutrition Revealed
Potassium Health Secrets Revealed

Stomach Remedies
Acid Reflux: Fast and Easy Cures For Acid Reflux
Asthma Treatment Cures With Remedies
How To Do Natural Colon Cleansing

Misc. Remedies
Effective Natural Hemorrhoids Treatment
Iron Deficiency Anemia

What Is A Hiatus Hernia
Best Varicose Vein Treatments?

Men's Health
Best Impotence Health Diet

Weight loss
Ten (10) Day Quick Success Weight Loss Program

To see all of the kindle books written by this author, go to this the Authors Profile Page or this URL:

http://tinyurl.com/b2f7wd3

If you need support or want to promote any of his e-books, please contact him at rss41@yahoo.com and expect a reply within 24 hours.

Give a Review

And, don't forget to give a review for this e-book at Amazon. It's not hard to give a review. It can be only a sentence or two. You don't have to leave a long review. A short review helps other people decide if they want to buy a book. So give a short review and give your thoughts to help other people and to help the author improve his book.

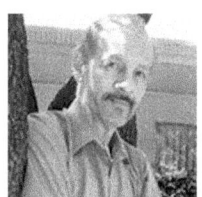

Here's to you for creating better health and living a long life.

Rudy Silva, Natural Nutritionist